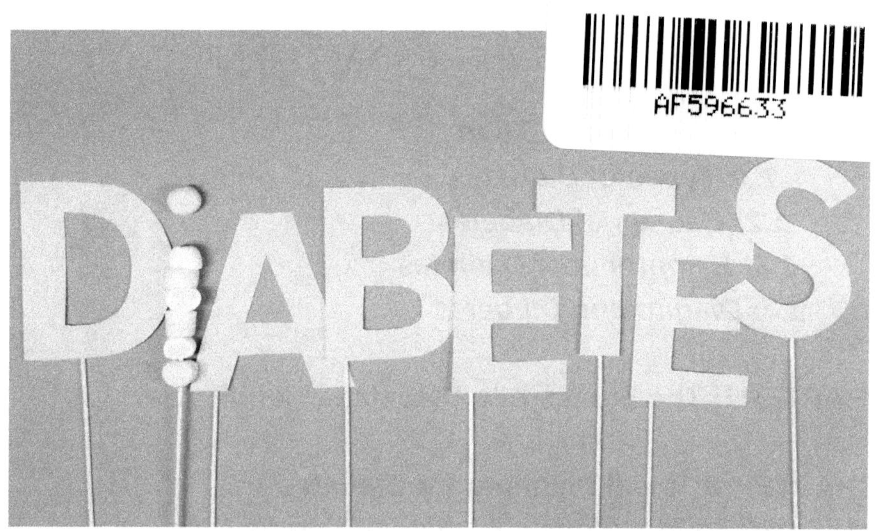

AND DIET

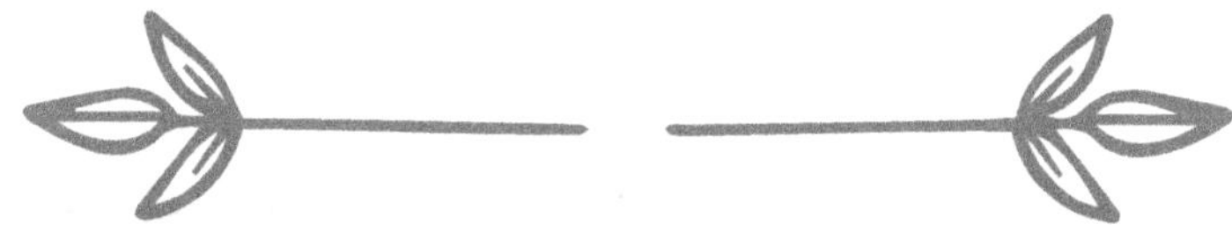

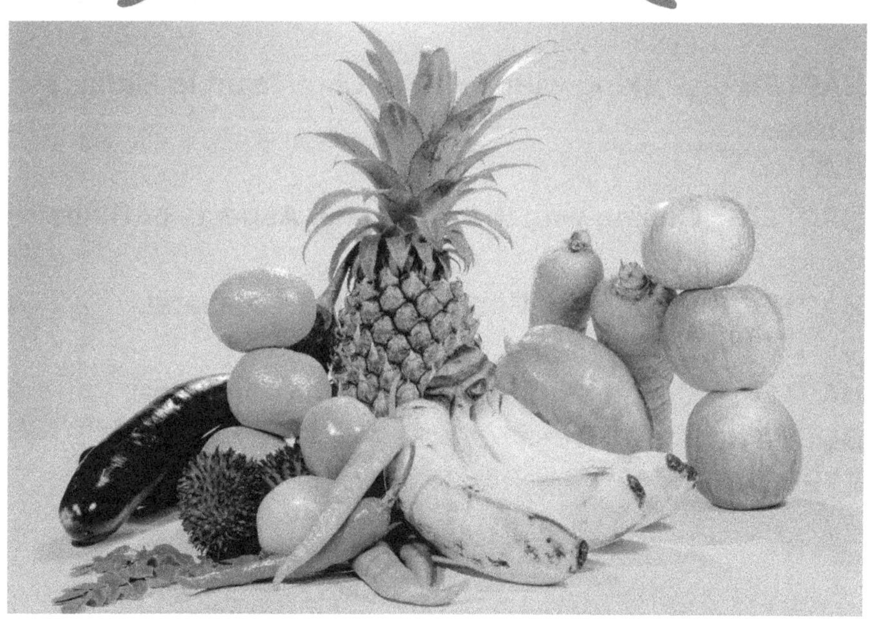

Author © Joseph Fawenu

2022

TABLE OF CONTENT

CHAPTER 1
INTRODUCTION

Diabetes is a chronic condition that affects the way the body processes blood sugar, or glucose. Glucose is the main source of fuel for the body, and it comes from the food we eat. In people with diabetes, the body either doesn't produce enough insulin (a hormone that helps regulate blood sugar) or it can't effectively use the insulin it does produce. This can cause high levels of sugar to build up in the blood, leading to a range of health problems if left untreated.

1.1 Types of Diabetes

There are two main types of diabetes: type 1 and type 2.

Type 1 diabetes is an autoimmune disease in which the body's immune system attacks and destroys the cells in the pancreas that produce insulin. This means that the body is unable to produce enough insulin to regulate blood sugar levels, and people with type 1 diabetes must take insulin injections or use an insulin pump to manage their condition.

Type 2 diabetes, on the other hand, is the most common form of diabetes. It occurs when the body becomes resistant to the effects of insulin or doesn't produce enough insulin to meet its needs. People with type 2 diabetes may be able to manage their condition with lifestyle changes, such as eating a healthy diet and exercising regularly, but some may also need to take oral medications or insulin injections to control their blood sugar levels.

There is also a third type of diabetes called **gestational diabetes**, which occurs during pregnancy. This form of diabetes usually goes away after the baby is born, but it increases the mother's risk of developing type 2 diabetes later in life.

1.2 Causes of Diabetes

The exact causes of diabetes are not fully understood, but a combination of genetic and environmental factors is thought to play a role. **In type 1 diabetes**, the body's immune system attacks and destroys the cells in the pancreas that produce insulin. This is thought to be triggered by a combination of genetic and environmental factors, such as viruses or other infections.

In type 2 diabetes, the body becomes resistant to the effects of insulin or doesn't produce enough insulin to meet its needs. This can be caused by a combination of factors, including a sedentary lifestyle, being overweight or obese, and a family history of diabetes.

Gestational diabetes is caused by hormonal changes during pregnancy, which can make it more difficult for the body to use insulin effectively. This can lead to high blood sugar levels during pregnancy.

1.3 Symptoms of Diabetes

The symptoms of diabetes can vary depending on the type of diabetes and how well the condition is managed. Some common symptoms of diabetes include:

- Increased thirst
- Frequent urination
- Fatigue
- Blurred vision
- Slow-healing wounds or infections
- Numbness or tingling in the hands or feet
- Unexpected weight loss

If you experience any of these symptoms, it's important to talk to your doctor. They can help determine if you have diabetes and develop a treatment plan to manage your condition.

1.4 Diagnosing Diabetes

To diagnose diabetes, your doctor will ask about your medical history and symptoms and conduct a physical exam. They may also recommend one or more of the following tests to measure your blood sugar levels:

I. A fasting blood sugar test, which measures your blood sugar after you have fasted for at least 8 hours.

II. An oral glucose tolerance test, which measures your blood sugar after you have fasted and then again 2 hours after you drink a sugary drink.

III. A hemoglobin A1C test, which measures your average blood sugar levels over the past 2-3 months.

Based on the results of these tests, your doctor can determine if you have diabetes and, if so, what type. They can then work with you to develop a treatment plan to manage your condition.

CHAPTER 2
The Basics of a Diabetes-Friendly Diet

Diet is an important part of managing diabetes. Eating a healthy, balanced diet can help you control your blood sugar levels and prevent complications of diabetes.

A diabetes-friendly diet is a balanced and nutritious diet that includes a variety of foods from all food groups. It should be tailored to your individual needs and preferences, and should be based on your age, activity level, and overall health.

Some general guidelines for a diabetes-friendly diet include:

I. Eating plenty of fruits, vegetables, whole grains, and legumes

II. Choosing lean proteins, such as fish, poultry, and plant-based proteins

III. Limiting or avoiding foods and drinks that are high in added sugars, sodium, and unhealthy fats

IV. Drinking plenty of water

V. Eating regular meals and snacks to help keep your blood sugar levels stable.

In addition, people with diabetes should pay attention to the amount and type of carbohydrates they eat, as well as the timing of their meals.

Carbohydrates are the main source of glucose in the diet, and they can have a big impact on your blood sugar levels. By eating carbohydrates in moderation and choosing complex carbohydrates, such as whole grains and starchy vegetables, over simple carbohydrates, such as sugary drinks and sweets, you can help keep your blood sugar levels within a healthy range.

It's important to work with a registered dietitian to develop a meal plan that is right for you. A registered dietitian can help you create a plan that includes the right balance of nutrients and fits your lifestyle.

CHAPTER 3
Meal Planning for Diabetes

Meal planning is an important part of managing diabetes. A good meal plan can help you control your blood sugar levels and maintain a healthy weight.

When planning your meals, it's important to include a variety of nutritious foods from all food groups. This means eating a balance of fruits, vegetables, whole grains, lean proteins, and healthy fats. It's also important to limit or avoid foods that are high in added sugars, sodium, and unhealthy fats.

Here are some tips for meal planning with diabetes:

I. Choose foods that are high in fiber, such as fruits, vegetables, whole grains, and legumes. Fiber can help slow down the absorption of sugar in the bloodstream, which can help keep your blood sugar levels stable.

II. Include protein with each meal and snack. Protein can help slow down the absorption of carbohydrates, which can help keep your blood sugar levels stable. Good sources of protein include lean meats, poultry, fish, eggs, and plant-based proteins such as beans and lentils.

III. Limit or avoid foods and drinks that are high in added sugars, such as soda, candy, and sweetened beverages. These foods can cause your blood sugar levels to spike quickly.

IV. Choose healthy fats, such as avocado, olive oil, and nuts. These fats can help you feel fuller for longer and can also provide essential nutrients.
V. Drink plenty of water. Staying hydrated can help your body function properly and can also help you feel full.

VI. Plan ahead and prepare meals in advance, when possible. This can help you avoid making unhealthy food choices when you're short on time. It's also a good idea to work with a registered dietitian to develop a meal plan that's tailored to your specific needs. A registered dietitian can help you create a plan that includes the right balance of nutrients to help you manage your diabetes.

3.1 Foods to Include in a Diabetes-Friendly Diet

A diabetes-friendly diet should include a variety of nutritious foods from all food groups. Some examples of foods that can be included in a diabetes-friendly diet are:

I. Fruits: Choose fresh, frozen, or canned fruits (without added sugars) and include a variety of colors. Some examples are apples, bananas, berries, citrus fruits, and mangoes.

II. Vegetables: Choose fresh, frozen, or canned vegetables (without added sodium) and include a variety of colors and types. Some examples are leafy greens, bell peppers, carrots, tomatoes, and sweet potatoes.

III. Whole grains: Choose whole-grain bread, pasta, rice, and cereals that are high in fiber. Some examples are whole-wheat bread, brown rice, quinoa, and oatmeal.

IV. Lean proteins: Choose lean meats, poultry, fish, eggs, and plant-based proteins. Some examples are chicken breast, salmon, tofu, and lentils.

V. Healthy fats: Choose healthy fats, such as avocado, olive oil, and nuts. These fats can help you feel fuller for longer and can also provide essential nutrients.

It's important to work with a registered dietitian to develop a meal plan that is right for you and includes the right balance of nutrients. A registered dietitian can help you create a plan that fits your lifestyle and food preferences.

3.2 Foods to Limit or Avoid in a Diabetes-Friendly Diet

In a diabetes-friendly diet, it's important to limit or avoid foods that are high in added sugars, sodium, and unhealthy fats. Some examples of foods to limit or avoid are:

·**Foods and drinks that are high in added sugars:** These include soda, candy, and sweetened beverages. These foods can cause your blood sugar levels to spike quickly, which can be harmful if you have diabetes.
·**Processed foods:** These are often high in sodium,

added sugars, and unhealthy fats. Examples include packaged snacks, frozen meals, and canned soups.

·**Unhealthy fats:** These include trans fats and saturated fats, which are often found in fried foods, processed snacks, and baked goods. These fats can raise your cholesterol levels and increase your risk of heart disease.

·**Alcohol:** Alcohol can interfere with the body's ability to regulate blood sugar levels, so it's important to limit your intake if you have diabetes. If you choose to drink, do so in moderation and avoid mixing alcohol with sugary mixers.

It's important to work with a registered dietitian to develop a meal plan that is right for you and includes the right balance of nutrients. A registered dietitian can help you create a plan that fits your lifestyle and food preferences.

3.3 Tips for Dining Out with Diabetes

Dining out can be challenging if you have diabetes, but with a little planning, you can enjoy a meal at a restaurant without compromising your health. Here are some tips for dining out with diabetes:

Look for restaurants that offer healthy options
Many restaurants now offer menus that cater to people with dietary restrictions, such as diabetes. Look for restaurants that offer a variety of vegetables, lean proteins, and whole grains.

Plan ahead. Look at the restaurant's menu online before you go, and decide what you will order ahead of time. This can help you avoid making impulsive choices that may not be healthy.

Don't be afraid to ask for what you want. If a dish on the menu doesn't meet your dietary needs, don't be afraid to ask the waiter to make adjustments. For example, you can ask for sauce on the side, or for your vegetables to be steamed instead of fried.

Portion control is key. Restaurants often serve large portions, so be mindful of how much you eat. You can ask for a to-go container and take part of your meal home, or share a dish with a friend.

Drink water. Water is your best choice when dining out. Avoid sugary drinks, such as soda and sweetened iced tea, which can cause your blood sugar levels to spike.
With a little planning and some healthy choices, you can enjoy dining out while managing your diabetes.

3.4 Using Carbohydrate Counting to Manage Diabetes

Carbohydrate counting is a way of managing diabetes that focuses on the amount of carbohydrates in your meals and snacks. Carbohydrates are found in many foods, including fruits, vegetables, grains, and milk.

When you eat carbohydrates, your body breaks them down into glucose (sugar), which can raise your blood sugar levels.

By counting the number of carbohydrates you eat at each meal and snack, you can better manage your blood sugar levels. This can be especially helpful if you take insulin or other diabetes medications that work by lowering your blood sugar levels.

To start carbohydrate counting, you will need to:

I. Learn how many carbohydrates are in the foods you eat: You can find this information on the food label or by using a carbohydrate counting app or book.

II. Plan your meals and snacks: Choose foods that are high in carbohydrates, such as fruits, vegetables, and whole grains, and include them in your meals and snacks.

III. Keep track of your carbohydrate intake: Use a food diary or app to record the number of carbohydrates you eat at each meal and snack.

IV. Adjust your insulin or medication doses: If you take insulin or other diabetes medications, you may need to adjust your doses based on the number of carbohydrates you eat. Work with your doctor or diabetes educator to create a plan for adjusting your doses.

Carbohydrate counting can be a useful tool for managing your blood sugar levels and improving your overall health. It's a good idea to work with a registered dietitian to develop a meal plan that is right for you.

CHAPTER 4
Managing Blood Sugar Levels with Exercise

Exercise is an important part of managing diabetes. Regular physical activity can help you control your blood sugar levels, maintain a healthy weight, and reduce your risk of heart disease and other complications.
When you exercise, your muscles use glucose (sugar) for fuel. This can help lower your blood sugar levels, especially if you have type 2 diabetes. Exercise can also increase your sensitivity to insulin, which can help your body use glucose more effectively.
There are many different types of exercise that can be beneficial for people with diabetes, including:

I. Aerobic exercise: This type of exercise, also known as cardio, gets your heart rate up and can include activities such as walking, running, cycling, and swimming.

II. Strength training: This type of exercise helps build and maintain muscle mass. It can include activities such as lifting weights, using resistance bands, or doing body weight exercises.

III. Flexibility and balance exercises: These exercises can help improve your range of motion and balance, which can help prevent falls and other injuries. Examples include yoga, tai chi, and Pilates.

It's important to talk to your doctor before starting a new exercise program, especially if you have any health conditions. Your doctor can help you create a plan that is safe and effective for managing your diabetes.

CHAPTER 5
The Role of Medications in Managing Diabetes

Medications can be an important part of managing diabetes. These medications can help control your blood sugar levels and reduce your risk of complications.
There are several different types of medications that are used to treat diabetes, including:

- **Insulin**: This is a hormone that helps regulate your blood sugar levels. People with type 1 diabetes and some people with type 2 diabetes may need to take insulin injections or use an insulin pump.

- **Oral medications**: These are medications that you take by mouth. They can help your body use insulin more effectively or help your pancreas produce more insulin.

- **GLP-1 receptor agonists**: These medications can help your body produce more insulin and reduce the amount of glucose (sugar) that your liver makes. They are typically used in combination with other diabetes medications.

-

SGLT2 inhibitors: These medications help your body get rid of excess glucose through your urine. They are typically used in combination with other diabetes medications.

.

It's important to work with your doctor to determine the right medication plan for you. Your doctor will consider your age, overall health, and other factors when prescribing medications for your diabetes.

CHAPTER 6
Working with a Health Care Team to Manage Diabetes

Managing diabetes can be complex and requires a team approach. It's important to work with a group of healthcare providers who can help you manage your condition and prevent complications.
Your healthcare team may include:

- **A primary care doctor:** This is the doctor who provides your overall medical care. Your primary care doctor can help manage your diabetes, monitor your blood sugar levels, and prescribe medications as needed.

- **A registered dietitian:** A registered dietitian can help you create a healthy meal plan that is tailored to your needs and preferences. They can also provide education and support to help you make healthy food choices.

- **A diabetes educator:** A diabetes educator is a healthcare provider who has special training in diabetes management. They can provide education and support to help you manage your diabetes, including information about medications, exercise, and healthy living.

An endocrinologist: An endocrinologist is a doctor who specializes in the endocrine system, which includes the hormones that regulate your body's functions. An endocrinologist can provide specialized care for people with diabetes and other endocrine disorders.

Other specialists: Depending on your needs, your healthcare team may also include other specialists, such as an ophthalmologist (eye doctor), podiatrist (foot doctor), or cardiologist (heart doctor), a pathologist or medical laboratory technologist.

Working with a healthcare team can help you manage your diabetes and prevent complications. It's important to communicate openly with your healthcare providers and follow their recommendations for managing your condition.

CHAPTER 7
Coping with the Emotional Aspects of Diabetes

Living with diabetes can be challenging, both physically and emotionally. It's normal to experience a range of emotions, including frustration, anger, and fear. It's important to find healthy ways to cope with these emotions and manage the stress of living with diabetes.
Here are some tips for coping with the emotional aspects of diabetes:
·**Talk to someone:** It can be helpful to talk to a trusted friend or family member about your feelings. You can also talk to a therapist or counselor who can provide support and guidance for managing your emotions.

Join a support group: Many people find it helpful to connect with others who are living with diabetes. You can find support groups in your community or online that can provide emotional support and information about managing your condition.

Take care of yourself: Self-care is important for managing the emotional aspects of diabetes. This can include getting regular exercise, eating a healthy diet, and getting enough sleep. It can also include activities that you enjoy, such as hobbies or spending time with friends and family.

Seek help if needed: If you are struggling to cope with the emotional aspects of diabetes, it's important to seek help. Your healthcare team can provide support and refer you to resources that can help you manage your emotions and stress.

Living with diabetes can be difficult, but with the right support and coping strategies, you can manage your condition and maintain good emotional health.

CHAPTER 8
Preventing Complications of Diabetes

Diabetes can lead to a range of health complications if it is not managed properly. These complications can include heart disease, nerve damage, kidney damage, and vision loss.
To prevent complications of diabetes, it's important to manage your blood sugar levels and maintain a healthy lifestyle. This can include:

Following a healthy meal plan: A healthy meal plan can help you control your blood sugar levels and maintain a healthy weight. It should include a variety of nutritious foods from all food groups and be tailored to your individual needs and preferences.

Getting regular exercise: Exercise can help you control your blood sugar levels, maintain a healthy weight, and reduce your risk of heart disease and other complications. It's important to talk to your doctor before starting a new exercise program.

Taking your medications as prescribed: If you take insulin or other diabetes medications, it's important to take them as prescribed by your doctor. This can help control your blood sugar levels and prevent complications.

Monitoring your blood sugar levels: Regularly checking your blood sugar levels can help you monitor your diabetes and make any necessary adjustments to your meal plan, exercise, or medications.

Managing other health conditions: If you have other health conditions, such as high blood pressure or high cholesterol, it's important to manage these conditions to prevent complications of diabetes. Your healthcare team can provide support and guidance for managing your overall health.

By following a healthy lifestyle and managing your diabetes, you can prevent or delay the onset of complications. It's important to work with your healthcare team to develop a plan that is right for you.

CHAPTER 9

Conclusion: Living Well with Diabetes

Diabetes is a chronic condition that affects the way the body processes blood sugar (glucose). There are two main types of diabetes: type 1 and type 2. In type 1 diabetes, the body does not produce enough insulin, a hormone that helps regulate blood sugar levels. In type 2 diabetes, the body does not produce enough insulin or does not use it effectively.

Managing diabetes involves making changes to your diet and exercise habits, and taking medications as prescribed. A healthy lifestyle can help you keep your blood sugar levels under control and prevent or delay the onset of complications.

This includes following a healthy meal plan, getting regular exercise, taking your medications as prescribed, and monitoring your blood sugar levels. It's also important to work with a healthcare team that can provide support and guidance for managing your diabetes.

By following a healthy lifestyle and working with your healthcare team, you can live well with diabetes and prevent or delay the onset of complications.

ABOUT

Joseph Fawenu is the author of the book "Diabetes and Diet." He is married and received his education at Ladoke Akintola University of Technology in Ogbonoso, Nigeria, where he studied Medical Laboratory Science. He has held various leadership roles throughout his career, including President of the Christian Student Fellowship at Government Secondary School Lafiagi in 2000/2001, Class Pastor for Medical Laboratory Science students in 2012/2013 (2012/2013 SET), and President of the Student Fellowship at Victory Chapel from 2012-2014. Currently, he serves as the Publicity Secretary for the Association of Medical Laboratory Scientists of Nigeria's SBM Chapter in Lagos. In his free time, he enjoys reading, writing, and meditation.

FIRST NIBCARE LABORATORIES
5, SAVAGE STREET, OPP. FEDERAL FIRE SERVICE,
OYINGBO, LAGOS, NIGERIA
joseph4fawenu@gmail.com

DIABETES AND DIET
1st Edition

REFERENCES

American Diabetes Association. (2020). Standards of medical care in diabetes—2020. Diabetes Care, 43(Supplement 1). https://care.diabetesjournals.org/content/43/Supplement_1

National Institute of Diabetes and Digestive and Kidney Diseases. (2021). Types of diabetes. https://www.niddk.nih.gov/health-information/diabetes/overview/types-diabetes

World Health Organization. (2021). Diabetes. https://www.who.int/news-room/fact-sheets/detail/diabetes

Mayo Clinic. (2021). Diabetes diet: Create your healthy-eating plan. https://www.mayoclinic.org/diseases-conditions/diabetes/in-depth/diabetes-diet/art-20044295

American Diabetes Association. (2021). Meal planning for people with diabetes. https://www.diabetes.org/nutrition/meal-planning

National Institute of Diabetes and Digestive and Kidney Diseases. (2021). Exercise and physical activity. https://www.niddk.nih.gov/health-information/diabetes/overview/preventing-problems/exercise-physical-activity

REFERENCES

American Diabetes Association. (2021). Diabetes medications. https://www.diabetes.org/resources/diabetes-care/medication-management/diabetes-medications

Mayo Clinic. (2021). Diabetes management: How lifestyle, daily routine affect blood sugar. https://www.mayoclinic.org/diseases-conditions/diabetes/in-depth/diabetes-management/art-20047871

National Institute of Diabetes and Digestive and Kidney Diseases. (2021). Coping with the emotional aspects of diabetes. https://www.niddk.nih.gov/health-information/diabetes/overview/preventing-problems/coping-emotional-aspects

World Health Organization. (2021). Diabetes complications. https://www.who.int/news-room/fact-sheets/detail/diabetes-complications

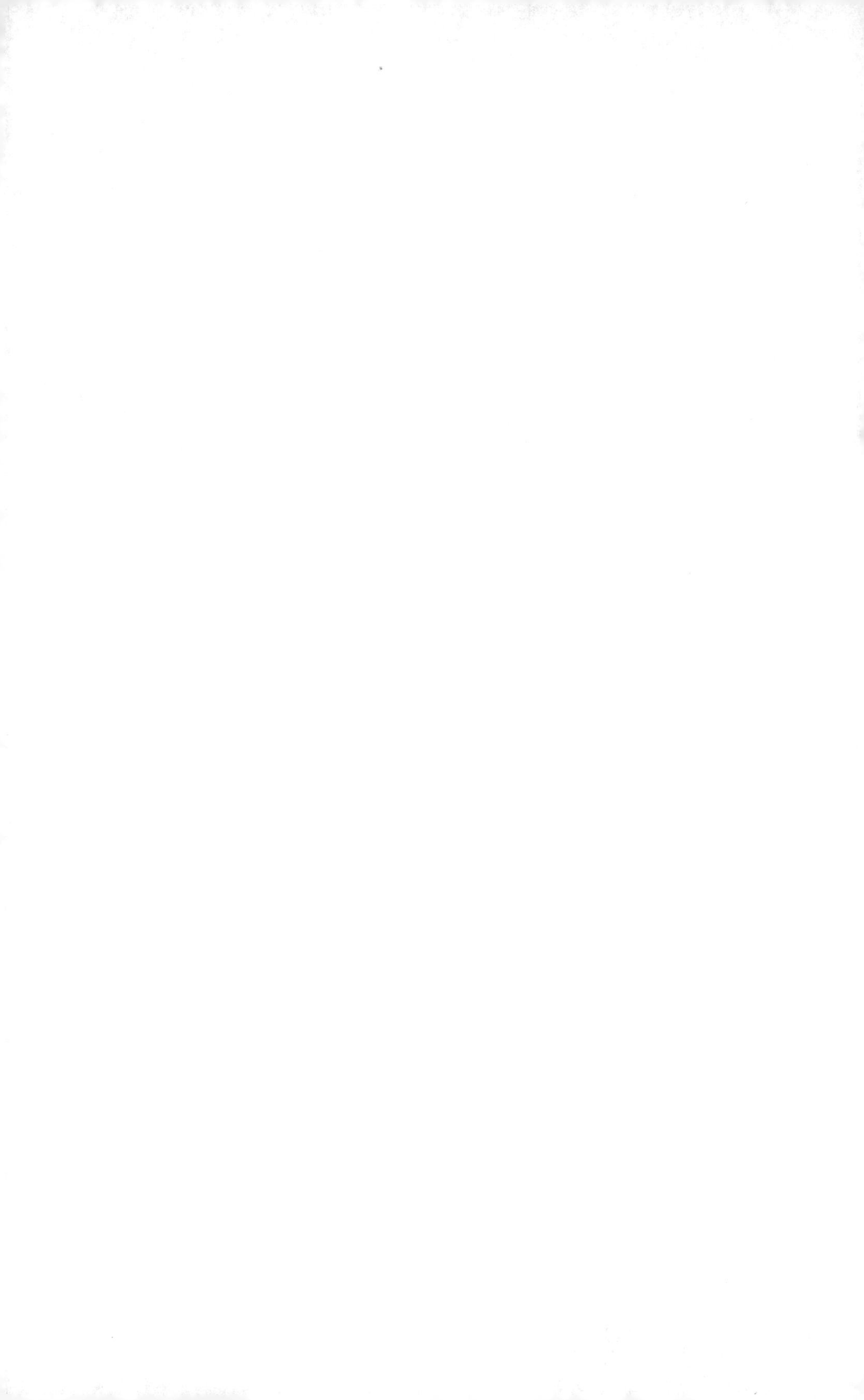

www.ingramcontent.com/pod-product-compliance
Lightning Source LLC
LaVergne TN
LVHW052112160826
845678LV00015B/3503

* 9 7 9 8 3 7 0 5 6 0 1 2 5 *